Faultless Diabetes: A Parent's Guide for a Juvenal Diabetic Child

By Sean M. Kinkaid

I0484162

Dedication:

To my Mother Marilyn, who taught me how to cook. And, Gales Creek Camp for Diabetic Children in Glenwood, Oregon.

Table of Contents

Forward

It happened again today and it's not your fault. A child was diagnosed with a condition although not common, is not rare. It can be the causation of a host of holy horrors not limited to: heart disease, stroke, blindness, depression, amputation and of course, death. The news that their child has this condition can be the cause of great anguish and suffering for the parent or parents. Many people experience enormous amounts of guilt and shame. The parent's condition is grief. The child's condition is diabetes. Juvenal diabetes.

I was there you see.

It was the very day of my 9th birthday. I couldn't stop drinking and going to the bathroom to urinate. I was flushed and gaunt with a death-like pallor and sullen, sunken eyes. But what really frightened my mother was that I couldn't, or wouldn't, eat anything.

So off to our family clinic to see our doctor and in short order I was informed that my first birthday gift was a trip. A trip to the hospital. There I stayed for 10 days. That was March of 1972 and it was the beginning of my diabetic journey. I learned how to survive this condition through every ring I could jump. I've learned how to thrive and go beyond the limitations that this condition can cause. I have forty-two years of experience with this condition (you notice I don't refer to it as a disease) and my knowledge and experiences will be, I hope, of great service to you. You see, I bring something to the table that many doctors can't.

I know more about it than they do.

No, not beyond their grasps as doctors, but, beyond their experiences as people. Especially, young people. Children. I've lived it and I'm here to help you and your children thrive from my experience.

The purpose of this book is to educate and and give guidance to you and to give you the comfort that comes from knowledge. The knowledge that your children can (and will) live lives as good, if not better than their peers and the knowledge that the condition your child has is not their fault. Its not your fault.

It is no one's fault.

This is faultless diabetes.

This guide is intended for the parents of a Juvenal diabetic, but this can all apply to a type 2 diabetic child as well. The principles are almost the same, with the challenges of the type 1 condition being more involved and difficult. The main difference being the injection of insulin vs. oral medication. Indeed, most modern day physicians refer to Juvenal diabetes as type 1, or insulin dependent and reject the notion that one must be a juvenile to contract this condition or that one must be an adult to contract type 2 or adult onset diabetes. These two lines have been blurred lately, so both conditions are addressed. Both are diabetic conditions and your child has it. This book is here to help. A parent need not be afraid. With the skills gained in this book a parent can go forward confidently and alleviate their child's worries and fears as well.

 What this book is not is a day- by- day instructional manual. There are plenty of those available. The basic mechanics of how to test blood sugars and draw insulin injections should be carried out in the proper venue. A book is no substitute for a quality diabetic camp or a physician's training session.

What this book deals with is the aspects that DON'T get discussed and dealt with. The human cost of diabetes and how to stop this condition from becoming a disease, robbing you and your child of happiness and peace of mind. I'm here to show you the ropes.

Chapter One - What is Diabetes?

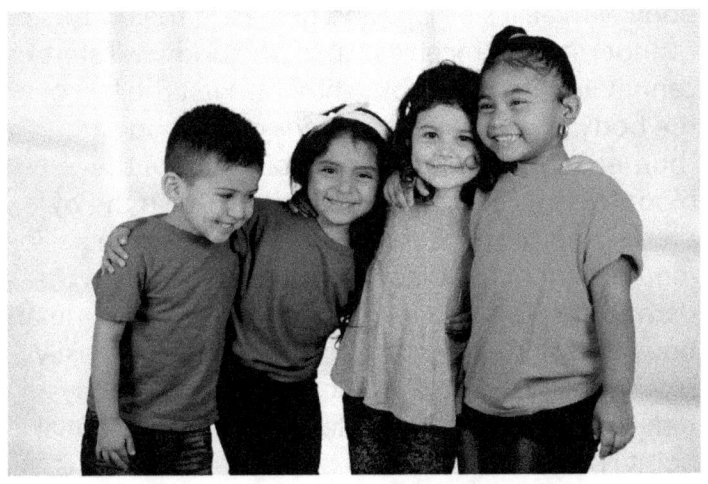

Diabetes mellitus is the condition of the organ the pancreas to not produce and regulate the hormone insulin. If the body has either produced insulin in a limited capacity (type 2) or it must be injected due to the body's inability to produce insulin at all, (type 1) then the body is in a diabetic condition. Type 2 is mentioned first because it is far more common than type 1 diabetes.

The essential purpose of insulin is two-fold. One, to break down the food consumed by the body from complicated carbohydrates, fats and proteins into a simple sugar (glucose) that can be assimilated in the body's cells. Two, the opening of these cells so that blood sugar and oxygen can enter and carbon dioxide can be expelled. Both of these functions are crucial for the human body to operate. Take away or restrict these actions and the body will rapidly start to deteriorate. This breakdown affects the entire body with all it's organs and tissues. If the body cannot make or receive insulin, the body will start to cannibalize itself for nourishment. First the fats of the body, then the lean proteins of the body are "burned". This causes a rapid poisoning of the bloodstream called keto-acidosis, wherein the by-product of this self consumption changes the basic metabolism of the diabetic and starts them on the path to sickness and if untreated, death. The human body is designed to not starve to death very easily, so, this mechanism is in place, however, it is only a temporary fix to stave off starvation. The essential point is that diabetes must be treated or death is assured. This may also explain why so many type 2 people have had terrible complications and premature death because-

THEY DIDN'T KNOW THEY HAD IT.

The slow regression of depleted amounts of insulin and the diabetic's inability to absorb and process insulin (insulin resistance) is the major reason that diabetes is so tragic and fatal for people of any age.

The upside for a Juvenal diabetic (type 1) is that the onset of the condition is so rapid and dramatic, such as mine, they end up in an ER or a doctor's clinic within a day or two of the onset. This can save their lives. It also means that the Juvenal diabetic is spared all of the complications that arise from a gradual decline in insulin production. In other words, your child has a clean slate and both you and your child can forge ahead with the best outcomes for your child's future. There doesn't need to be complications if proper treatment is started.

Rejoice!

Juvenal diabetes may have just saved your child's life.

There are many factors that can lead to your child developing diabetes. The main factor is of course, genetics. Does Juvenal diabetes or adult onset diabetes run in your family? If so, then you and any offspring will have a predisposition to it as well. Your ethnic background is a factor as well. If you are of African, Hispanic or native American descent, then you are in a high risk group. The statistic for developing diabetes in children of diabetic parents is roughly 50%. Half. The recessive genes seem to play a large part of the genetic "crap shoot" that can determine a diabetic condition. The chances for non-diabetic parents with diabetes in their family to have JD children is unknown, but, the risk due to this predisposition is a warning that steps can be taken to lessen certain stresses to the body.

The primary strategy is three-fold; exercise, diet and stress reduction.

Indeed, the chief strategy for treating JD is the best way to prevent it. Greater detail will be given later in the book regarding these measures, but they still remain the cornerstones of proper diabetic and pre-diabetic care.

Major illnesses can also be the culprit to triggering the body into not producing insulin, such as what can happen in pregnancies or with heart attacks. High fevers and even traumatic events can create the condition in the body that results in either a partial or total breakdown in the pancreas's ability to produce insulin.

The point?
Try as you might to prevent your child from developing diabetes, you can't stop it. You can't control the weather, or time, or your child getting the flu. You can try, but if they do get ill and it leads to JD, you are not at fault, just as you are not at fault for anything genetic you were born with. It's the human condition. You did not "curse" your child to a life of doom. You gave your child life.

Your child is looking to you for strength and guidance. Please remember that your attitude regarding your child's JD will have a direct effect on that child's attitude. If you project impatience or negativity, your child will develop the same mental attitudes concerning their condition. This leads to the trouble I am trying to stop with this book.

YOU are more important to your child's short and long term health than any doctor.

This is why information is so important. You must become an expert in JD, so your child can become one. If you slack off and become indifferent, then you will see the same attributes in your child.
  Be the rock they need for stability and they can be your rock as well. It's a team effort. Remember, you lead the team.

Chapter Two - What are the Effects that JD has on the Brain and Emotions?

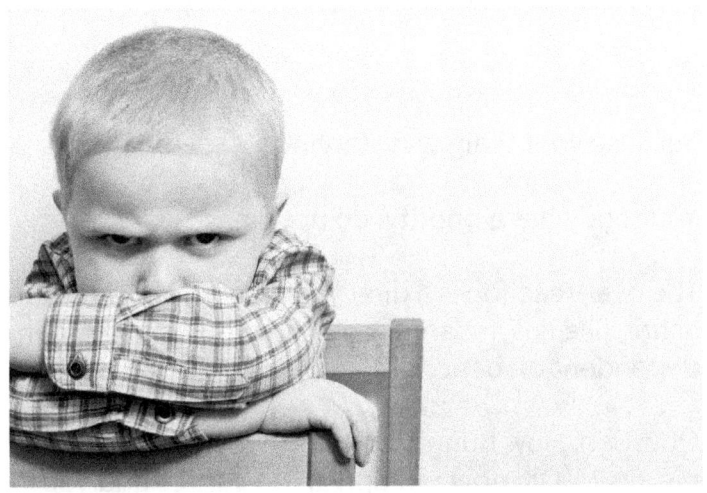

Answer. Plenty.

The results of bad blood-sugar control are everywhere. Road rage, air rage and people exploding with inappropriate anger are, in the author's opinion, the direct result of LOW-blood-sugar (hypoglycemia). When the brain, the organ, receives too little glucose or oxygen, the other crucial component in proper brain function, the body will go into "fight or flight" response and the adrenal gland will flood the bloodstream with hormones that cause agitation. The mind becomes too foggy to respond, because the brain is struggling to remain conscious and civil.

Have you ever had a reservation to a restaurant and they were taking too long to either seat or serve you and you were really hungry? How did you react? With 4-letter words and lots of snarling?

Why?

Because your brain was starving.

Your body has a priority: do not die.

The over-reaction is a direct result of the body acting like it is in danger, which, if you are an insulin dependent diabetic, it is.

Question. How hungry do you have to be to "feel" hungry? " OK. now multiply that by three and you will come close to understanding what a JD feels when they "get hungry'".

With a insulin dependent diabetic, (JD) the starvation factor is no joke. The plunging blood sugar levels can lead to unconsciousness. If that diabetic is not treated with oral glucose or an injection of the hormone glucagon, they will go into a coma and then permanent brain damage results. Then death. The most horrifying aspect of JD is that; passing out and being left to die. Long term management is crucial for diabetic care, but nothing is more of a threat to your child's life than hypoglycemia.

DOCTORS DON"T WARN ABOUT THIS ENOUGH.

They focus on high blood-sugar (hyperglycemia) and underplay the low blood-sugar dangers. Please take it from me. I have 42 years experience living with this condition. Learning how to spot low blood-sugars in your child is essential to proper care.

For the brain to operate properly, it must have ample oxygen and glucose. These two factors are crucial in mood and emotional stability.

When your child takes their morning insulin injection, they are now committed to that shot. They cannot un-inject themselves. Thus, once that insulin is entering the bloodstream, the body must be fed a meal that combined with the insulin, allow energy to created and used in movement, exercise or even the most basic bodily functions. This is the balance.

If, by chance, they miss breakfast they will be going into a state of low blood-sugar rapidly and this is called an "insulin reaction'" A state in which the body starts the fight or flight reaction in the brain and the shutting down of the body's unnecessary systems to stave off unconsciousness. Before an insulin reaction occurs, a diabetic will experience what I call "falling fast". That means the mental and emotional tasks start to become difficult and your energy level noticeably drops.

The symptoms of an insulin reaction are very important for you, the parent, to watch for and recognize. In it's milder onset a "reaction" may feel like being tired or sleepy, drowsy, confused, irritable, surly or just upset. This usually happens when your child is active (we will revisit that later) or it's right before mealtime.

These insulin reactions can easily be treated with fruit juice or other foods high in sugars, either natural or not. As previously explained, these sugary foods are broken down into the simpler sugar, glucose, which is assimilated rapidly in the bloodstream. Within minutes, your child will start to perk up and will be ready to eat the meal intended.

Caution!

Do not try and give your child regular foods which are not high in sugars if the insulin reaction is severe. The foods cannot be broken down into glucose fast enough for the body and the child's blood-sugar will continue to plummet. It is actually possible for a JD to lapse into unconsciousness from low blood-sugar with a stomach full of food.

If a mild insulin reaction is not treated quickly the symptoms become worse. These include sweating, shaking, dizziness, rapid pulse, breathing heavy, lack of feeling in your fingers, hands, toes and feet, diminished sight and hearing and the inability to resolve a decision or mental task. In essence, your mental and physical "plug" has been pulled and the life force in you is draining out. This can be serious. Many diabetic children have whats referred to as a "brittle condition" and they are prone to very rapid losses of glucose, also, they often have the diminished ability to recognize the symptoms of low blood-sugar fast enough. A parent must know what to expect and how to supervise a JD who is brittle. They can have a much greater propensity to lapse into unconsciousness much faster than a non-brittle diabetic.

A tell-tale sign that a JD is about to pass out is the blank and unblinking stare they give you. Their eyes glaze over and they look like they are sleep walking. Then, they go under. If your child is diagnosed as brittle, then you must be just that more diligent in that child's treatment and care. They require you to be more regimented on a daily basis.

The most important thing to understand is that your diabetic child is under a tremendous amount of emotional stress that you might not be aware of. The human brain is affected by blood-sugar levels and much of it is in plain sight. But, the private tensions are deeper and are directly related to the body trying to reach balance while coping with a condition that changes their ability to feel "balanced". It's a roller-coaster and you and your child need to work together so the ride is a lot less scary.

Also, please remember to be a little more gentle with diabetic children. They might be more "emotional" than other children. This is normal and is in step with the condition.

Chapter Three
Depression in Diabetic Children

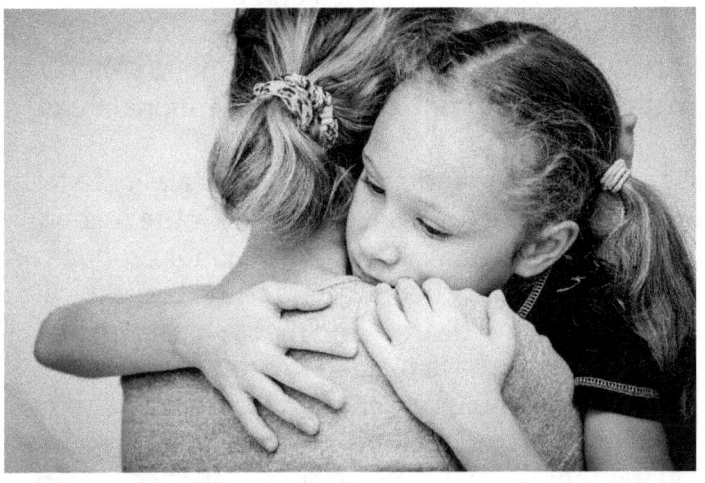

Diabetes can rob people of certain abilities and the one issue I never hear discussed enough is this: depression.

I am not a doctor, so I make this statement as a well informed and intended layperson. There is what I call, The "Triangle of Despair'" with depression at on corner and obesity and diabetes at the other two corners. There seems to be a direct correlation between theses three factors that are hormone related and give us a clue about diabetes. The bodies ability to cope with stress is the unifying factor in my theory.

When the human body is under stress, the amount of blood-sugar rises and stays elevated until the stress is relieved. This is difficult enough for a non diabetic, but especially hard on a JD. The elevation of blood-sugars creates the imbalances in the body's ability to correct itself and the diabetic condition becomes uncontrollable. If elevated blood-sugars remain high, then the mind suffers the inability to cope with mental and emotional tasks.

As I previously mentioned, the body's ability to take in oxygen and expel carbon-dioxide is the second crucial roll of insulin. If the body cannot produce or assimilate insulin, then the cells of the brain start to break down and distress and mental upset ensues. The brain must have oxygen to process the vast amount of stimulus entering the mind. Long term mismanagement of blood-sugars almost guarantees mental depression in diabetics. Again, it's a chicken or the egg scenario of which came first- the depression or the diabetes.

In combination with obesity, you have again, The Triangle of Despair.

However, please take comfort that the depression is very treatable and if diabetic related (not clinical depression or other mental conditions not associated with diabetes) can be corrected with increased care to lower blood-sugars and reduce stresses to the mind and body that exacerbate this depressed condition.

I myself developed clinical depression at age five. Then, in concert with my diabetes, it created within me a strong disposition for a depressed state in general. This drags down one's metabolism and creates the basis for insulin resistance. A diabetic's main weapon to combat high-blood-sugar is also the main way to address depression; exercise, and more exercise.

Exercise

Indeed, I would like to take this opportunity to say this.

Your diabetic child must learn to be an athlete.

Not a professional one, but a gifted and dedicated amateur for the rest of their lives. Keeping their body's in great physical shape will make your child's diabetic management possible. Without consistent exercise, the opposite is true. You will not be able to manage their condition.

In the old days, say the 40's to the 70's, this was the main focus of diabetic care and it was very effective. But, with the rise of sugar consumption, sedentary lifestyles, increases in stress and inadequate PE in schools, has created a desperate need to return to this old principle;

Be active.

I recommend that a JD do some activity or movement (walking is great) after every meal. This will slow down the assimilation of the foods eaten and distribute blood-sugar to the major and minor muscle groups. This helps immensely in allowing the meal to be digested with the help of the insulin levels being high enough to allow breaking down the food into, again, glucose. Diabetics in general are prone to feeling "logey" after eating. This is a cue to move and exercise. As your child becomes more acclimated to this athleticism, you will notice a return of energy and mental acuity that the JD condition was hindering. They will have "snap" in their step and plenty of enthusiasm for life. In other words, the opposite of depression.

Nutrition

The second tier of dealing with diabetic depression is nutrition.

The foods that a diabetic child eats can be the main reasons for lack of energy and focus. Foods that are high on the glycemic index scale such as sugars, starches and fruits, spike the body's insulin requirements far faster than a JD's body can cope with this need. Thus, a dwindling return effect happens. The other foods that are slower to assimilate such as proteins and fats are hindered by the diabetic's lack of insulin, which again, is necessary to break foods down. High blood-sugars hinder the whole process of food breakdown and digestion. The food ingested will simply be eliminated as best the body can, with no ability to gain nourishment or calories. This is why poor control affects the bowels and digestion in general of diabetics. But, again, it is preventable by proper blood-sugar control.

The best diet is one that fuels your child's body for the amount of "work" or activity they may need to do. If your child is active daily, they may consume far more carbohydrates than a more sedentary child. The response that child has to the foods they eat will give you a chance to make the changes they require in their diet. A high protein/ fat diet with low sugar and starch is best suited for diabetics in general. This is also the best way to contain the factors that lead to depression. Your child's insulin requirements won't spike and they will also be far less prone to the effects of low blood-sugar mental upsets. This combination will start your child back to better emotional health by removing the chemical turmoil that these blood-sugar issues create.

Of course, a person's life is far more complicated than that, but few people outside of Juvenal diabetics and hypoglycemics (the condition of producing excess insulin) know what havoc poor blood-sugar control has for taking away one's emotional base.

Do not listen to the old food pyramid nonsense about heavy grain and dairy consumption. For a diabetic, these two foods should not be a staple of their diets. All grains are carbohydrates. Lactose is the sugar from milk products. It is high on the glycemic index and thus should be limited.

High carbohydrate and sugar consumption, even with fats and proteins will lead directly to that dreaded roller coaster effect that we all want to avoid.

Diets high in Omega-3 fatty acids can also stabilize mood. Fish, nuts and legumes are an excellent source. Most dietitians would also agree to limit your child's intake of red meat and processed luncheon meats as well. Stick to meats such as chicken, turkey, pork and seafood.
 Don't miss any opportunity to introduce vegetable proteins in every form.

This in combination with fats strongly assists in repairing the damages to the bodies tissues. Most germane to our subject; brain and nerve tissues. For a diabetic, this is even more important due to the higher sugar content in their blood. Diabetics heal more slowly than normal people because of this. A great diet, along with proper amounts of hydration and sleep, will regenerate your child's body and let them catch up to their non-diabetic peers.

Fresh fruits and vegetables are also essential for energy and hydration as well as their nutritional benefits. Always substitute these instead of sugars or even grains or starches. They help minimize inflammation in the muscles and joints. Indeed, try to avoid wheat. It is not suitable to a diabetic because of the high glycemic index and gluten. Even if a diabetic person is not gluten intolerant, it is better to stay clear of wheat products because of the insulin requirements. Again, any simple carbohydrate will spike the insulin needed by the body. Thus, by avoiding these "spike" foods, your child will have the ability to stabilize their blood-sugars and with it, their moods.

Remember, that all carbohydrates turn into glucose, so limit them to one-third of your child's diet with the corresponding fats and proteins making up the balance. Fructose is the sugar from fruits and some vegetables, so limit these foods to when the body is going to be active, is best.
Example. The first thing a diabetic child should eat in the morning is fruit, either juice or whole. it is best for their digestion and raising their blood-sugar levels that usually will have lowered during sleep.

After exercise is also a good time for a fruit snack. Most people, diabetic or not, eat fruit as the last course or desert. This is a mistake. Fruit is best consumed on an empty stomach because fruit is not digested in the stomach, it is digested first in the duodenum. Then, the small intestines. This is why you will taste cantaloupe long after eating it last at a brunch. It can't make it to the duodenum and gets caught at the top of your digestive system. For a diabetic, eating it first will, again, raise their blood-sugar, but not spike it, priming the body for the longer lasting foods. This is the key.

No spikes.

Any spikes in glucose requires a dramatic raise in insulin requirements. Which is more than your diabetic child can physically accomplish.

It's that simple.

The game plan is to avoid the hills and the valleys. The highs and the lows of blood-sugar and insulin.

This is the foundation to a healthy mood and mindset.

A healthy, functioning brain. Free from distress and sugar related upset.

Nutritional supplements are highly recommended, especially the essential metals such as zinc, chromium and Iron. These metals assist in the absorption of insulin. Large amounts of both water and oil soluble vitamins should be a part of your child's daily diet . B and E vitamins are great for mood control, especially krill oil. They are of course, supplemental to a nutritious diet, not a substitute. I also highly recommend digestive enzymes, even for children. Anything that assists the digestive process is a plus for diabetics. They also will reduce the effects of lactose intolerance, even with small amounts of dairy that is consumed. Many foods have milk solids and other hidden dairy additives. Digestive enzymes, along with plenty of water, exercise and proper diet will ensure regularity and proper bowel health as well. One less thing to be stressed about.

Hydration is also part of this equation. A diabetic should be drinking fresh, clean water all day long. It should be the principal liquid your JD child drinks. Avoid making fruit drinks or other sweetened drinks staples of your diabetic's diet.

They are full of calories, spikes your child's need for insulin and take a great deal of water to process. Plenty of water allows the kidneys to eliminate extra sugar that "spills" into the urine. Constant hydration keeps the kidneys functioning properly and keeps the large intestine (the largest deposit of water in the body) properly filled, which again, is the foundation for proper elimination.

Proper hydration serves another key role that affects a diabetic's mood: blood pressure. Mental acuity and all other physical functions are affected by blood pressure as well as blood sugar. Drinking plenty of water keeps the whole body in balance and assists in all of the ways that are good for your diabetic child.

Stress relief

The third component of combating diabetic depression is stress relief and management. Now were going into the heart of the matter. If stress runs up blood-sugar, then all efforts must be made to prevent stress. Quite a tall order, But we have already addressed two of these strategies: diet and exorcise. Both actively start a person on the proper road for stress reduction in the body. What about the mind?

Like my advise about being an athlete, your Juvenal diabetic child must become organized and dedicated to an active social and professional life. They need to be engaged in the world and the people within it. Isolation is not conducive to this. Video games and social media are high stress, with no activity. Team activities are the opposite. Team sports, drama, dance, hiking with friends, or any other thing that is an active outlet for their stress reduction. It's being around others that is the stress reducer. Now their minds can connect with other minds and they will find they have much of the same issues in common with their non diabetic friends. Then they will forget about their diabetes and start focusing on being kids. The friends they make will learn how to be there for them without treating them as different.

Now we get to conflicts. The blood-sugar roller coaster effect can be caused by the stresses we get from other people. Learning social skills will be most important to avoiding conflicts with others and coping with the emotions of others, without being directly affected themselves. This also means they must constantly be aware of the negative personality types who will engage them in emotional drama and turmoil. As always with diabetics, it's a balancing act. Good structure with plenty of social interaction, combined with plenty of down time for proper rest and recovery. Your child must learn how to let the attitudes of others and their comments slide off their backs like water off a duck's back. They must become masters at avoiding personal upset.

Keep an active interest in your child's activities and friends. Talk to them about what may be bothering them if you notice they seem upset. Just talking about any problem will help alleviate their stress about it. Be their sounding board and and give them the support to help them solve the problems of life.

A good time to get together as a family and reduce stress is a family meal. This should be, for the whole family, a time of peace and relaxation. Try to avoid upsetting topics and conversations. Let this be a time of civilized interaction.

Something to remember. Diabetics are experiencing low blood-sugar before eating and will not be attentive, nor talkative. You can visibly see the color return to their faces as they eat.

So, don't take it wrong if they are not responsive before eating. They need fuel in order to think. After the meal they will be fully able to speak and interact normally. It is a night and day difference.

Sleep

Sleep is another important component of stress reduction for diabetics. The average person does not get their required sleep. The JD has no such luxury. They must have at least 8 hours a night. Nine would be even better. Again, healing of the body and mental recovery is the key here. Just as sugars in their bloodstream impedes healing, so does lack of sleep. It has also been determined that lack of sleep causes mental upset and irritability. Two things to be avoided by diabetics. Set a time for going to bed and, most importantly, a steady time to rise. This will help set their internal time-clocks and keep them in a consistent sleep cycle. This is just as important as any other factor in their diabetic control. So, please don't discount it.

Afternoon naps are also a great idea. This has been proven to positively affect the mental abilities of those who take them, diabetic or not. As a parent, you must see and know if your child is tired because of a long day or because of high blood-sugar. Being tired all the time is an indication of poor control. Be observant to your child's energy level and how well they are sleeping and where their blood-sugars are running.

Blood testing

Which brings us to blood testing. The only real way to manage diabetes is through constant blood testing. It is the best tool available to compare how a JD feels and what they are registering on their blood test. Trying to go by feel is a fool's errand. We all do it. We get lazy and lackadaisical. Testing should be an engrained habit. like insulin and food, it is always an essential component for a Juvenal diabetic to have their testing equipment handy.

The best time to test is anytime your child is uncertain about how much blood-sugar they have and in what direction that blood-sugar is going. Up or down. If your child tests twice in one hour they will know where they are in the insulin/ blood-sugar mix and can change their intake of either things. However, that is only when dialing in an insulin dosage with food and activity.
The normal system should be 10 minutes before meal times or snack times. Then check one hour after eating to see how high their blood-sugar elevated. If needed, test again after two hours. This will tell the whole story about how much activity, food and insulin your child requires, with NO guessing. After meal testing is the master key to managing your child's blood-sugars, and thus, their diabetes. Your child doesn't have to test these many times, everyday, but before and after all meals and bed-time is a must. It gives you, your child and your

doctor the clear records to fine-tune your child's condition.

This will help immensely in reducing stress in your JD child's life and remove the causes of diabetic depression. Remember, that letting you down or disappointing you as parents are a source of stress. Good control through testing eliminates that stress source and gives good evidence of a better level of health.

Anger in diabetics

Another aspect of diabetes that is seldom mentioned is anger. The natural anger that arises in anyone who has had their health compromised. It is a feeling of betrayal. That your body has abandoned or has forsaken you. plus, the inconvenience and discomfort. Many diabetic children will get depressed and start "cheating" on their diets and become obstinate and uncooperative. It is a normal reaction to this condition and as I've tried to demonstrate, it is reversible and treatable.

By being there as parents, you can see the changes and seek remedy to whatever is at cause for their anger. Sometimes kids (and adults) just get tired of being diabetic and being different. It isn't apparent most of the time that a child has JD or type 2 diabetes, so people don't understand why they have restrictions and barriers to what you can do.

Children don't like being the center of that kind of attention. It can single a child out, which most people don't want. As a diabetic, we encounter many individuals who should know something about diabetes, yet, the level of ignorance remains startling high. Imagine trying to explain that you are having an insulin reaction and that you need sugar immediately. I have had supposedly educated and bright people refuse to assist me when I had insulin reactions because, "diabetes means your allergic to sugar. I don't want to kill you!". Not quite. This level of ignorance can be fatal. It's enough to make a diabetic a little angry.

Also, there is is the anger that comes from professional loss. I for instance was far more depressed and affected by being told in the hospital, that I could not be in the military than having diabetes. All I wanted to do was be in the Air Force. Yes, I know many people say things at nine and they change their minds. But, I was very serious and had wanted to be in the Air Force since I was six. It wasn't the shots or the dietary restrictions or anything else related to the day by day aspects of my diabetes. It was the loss of my dream that hurt me the most. I lost my career on my ninth birthday. A not so happy birthday.

I was also told in short order that I could not be a commercial pilot as well. I could not be a firefighter, a cop, an EMT, an air traffic controller or even a forest ranger. I wouldn't be able to pass the physicals for any of these professions. Even in trades where I wasn't precluded, it is still an uphill climb to be hired compared to a healthy, thus, non-diabetic job applicant. Diabetes is one of the most expensive conditions a person can have. We require a great deal of care over (hopefully) a long life. Many companies shy away from extending health care coverage to people with life-long conditions. These are just some of the things that can frustrate your child, beyond just feeling different from most everyone else. Please don't overlook this, because it does affect children more than adults realize. Children and adults alike consider their vocations as their identity. Nobody feels good about losing their identity.

This is why gaining control of their life will help them to find the calling that will be their profession. Knowing what they can't do will change their expectations for a future profession. Hopefully, not in a negative way, but in a constructive fashion. Explore what they want to do and can do. That will help them make the transition from professional disappointment to professional triumph.

Your Depression

We have addressed your child, now we shall see how your doing.

How did you feel when your child was diagnosed with diabetes? Were you scared, angry or numb? Did you have dreams and hopes that were dashed when you got the news? Did you think about all the people that you have known and what their experiences with diabetes was, and felt despair? Did you get angry at your self, your spouse and or, your child?   Have you said out loud or in private,"what did we do to deserve this?!"   Congratulations, it's official. You are human.

It is perfectly natural to feel grief and loss. You love your child and you want to protect them. The hype surrounding diabetes is enough to scare anyone. Most of the books I have read in the last thirty years did more to discourage and frighten me than instructing or inspiring me to good health. These books make it seem that your fate is sealed and that you should resign yourself to poor health and a diminished quality of life. They even call diabetes a disease, not a condition , as I do. As my first paragraph said. "It's a host of holy horrors". That's what the "experts" would have you believe. It doesn't have to be that way.

Don't let them spook you. Here's one reason why.

When I was laying in my hospital bed feeling sorry for myself forty-two years ago, my nurse came in and told me the truth.

I was the luckiest kid in that hospital.

She told me that life is like a carnival wheel. and that we as humans, have to occasionally take a spin. She told me that it was my turn and the wheel was called injury, sickness or death.

She informed me that their were children who would never walk again, or see or ever get to go home. They were going to die, there in that hospital. "You don't have cancer, or were injured for life in a traffic accident. You didn't suffocate or near drown and need hospital care for the rest of your life. You spun the wheel and all you got was diabetes. You won the spin. You lucked out."

You as parents won the spin too. As I have tried to show you, diabetes is not a death sentence. It's just a condition. When you allow diabetes to be unchecked and untreated, then, it is a disease. Stay on top of it and your child may actually be healthier than their friends and classmates. You win again.

Your child will be able to do most everything a non-diabetic can. They just can't produce insulin, which in the grand scheme, is not a tragedy. Please realize this and take comfort from it. There are indeed, far worse things that could have happened.

Chapter Four
Weight Loss for Diabetic Children

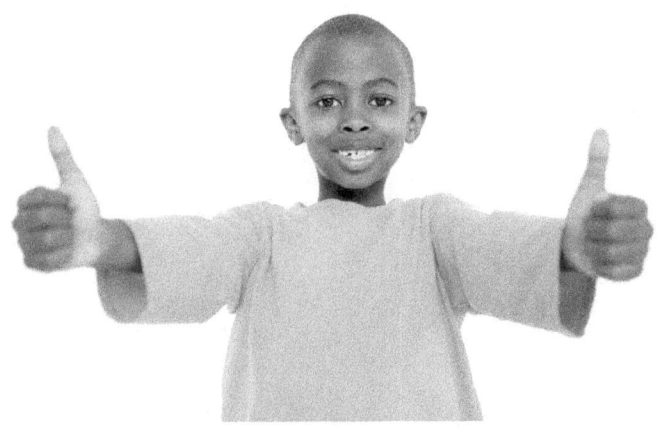

This is going to be a short chapter. The best way to lose fat and maintain proper weight is to follow what I have already written. This is the last corner of The Triangle of Despair. Exercise, low sugar/starch diet and stress reduction and the weight will fall off. Naturally.

An important fact is the body can absorb insulin much better when the body is at proper weight. Many type 2 diabetics cured themselves with weight reduction. It cured their insulin resistance. A type 1 diabetic who is obese will shed their weight and the need for more insulin, which accounts for the body to gain excess fat in the first place. Yes, excess insulin creates fat in the body. Furthermore, a JD will feel a lot better about themselves being at proper weight, thus, less depression. That is how your diabetic child will defeat The Triangle of Despair.

Chapter Five
FAQs

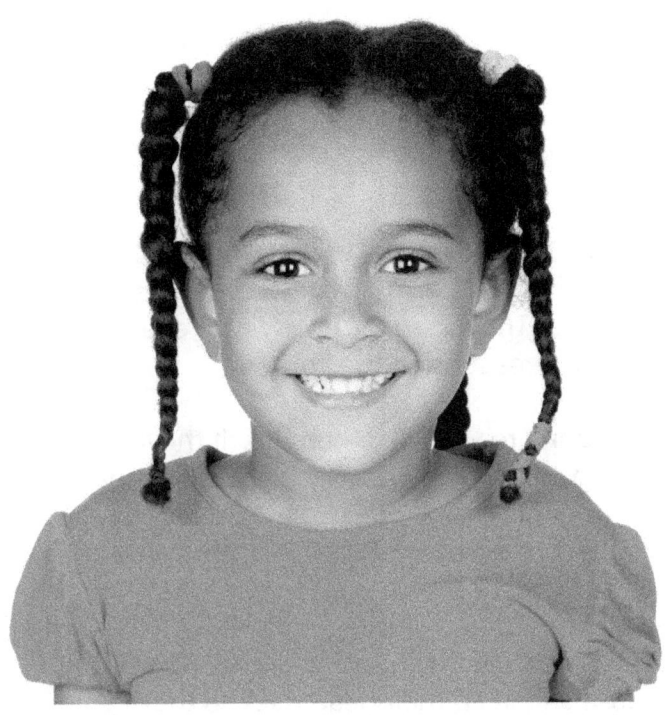

Question: What sport(s) is best for a diabetic child?

Answer: The best sports are basketball, soccer, track, volleyball, cross training, bike riding and the number one exercise. Swimming. These are great for both cardio and strength/endurance training. Try to avoid contact sports such as football, wrestling and boxing or contact martial arts. The healing factor is the reason. Plus, infections are minimized with less contact. This doesn't mean that contact sports are out, but extreme caution must be taken to avoid injuries.

Question: My child is brittle and I worry about low blood-sugars in the night. How do I know if my child is having an insulin reaction in their sleep?

Answer: Get a flashlight, one with the old bulbs, not an LED, and shine the light on your child's face while they sleep. They should turn away or even put a hand up in reaction to the light.

If they don't react, wake them up. If they don't wake up, they are in extreme low blood sugar. You must administer oral glucose by placing the glucose on the inside of their mouth, between the cheek and gums.

Rub the sides of the mouth to assist in melting the glucose and keep their head back so they can swallow the glucose. When they awaken treat their reaction with more sugary foods.

The best way to avoid early morning low blood-sugars to give your child a bedtime snack such as crackers and peanut-butter.

This snack is optimal, because it has protein, fat and carbohydrate in the same feeding. This will sustain them through the long night. Make sure that your child brushes and flosses afterward, so give them the snack a half-hour or so, before actual "bedtime'" If by chance, they have a digestive issue, then prepare the snack one full hour before they lay down to sleep.

Question: How do I protect my JD child from vision problems?

Answer: Follow all of the previously mentioned actions to gain control over your child's blood-sugars. High blood sugar (hyperglycemia) is the main cause of deleted eyesight and blindness in diabetics. The retina will start to "starve" of oxygen and begin a chemical process that creates new blood vessels to supply oxygenated blood to the retina.

This is called diabetic retinopathy. These new blood vessels are weak and easily ruptured. This causes bleeding into the eye (vitriol hemorrhage) which blocks out the light supply to the retina and the optic nerve, restricting eyesight.

If these new blood vessels continue to grow and hemorrhage they create a tugging (vitriol traction) on the retina which can tear or even detach the retina. This is very serious and if not successfully corrected with micro-surgery, can cause the retina to fully detach from the optic nerve, which presently, causes total and irreversible blindness.

Cataracts (discoloration and fogging of the eyes lens) are also a problem with diabetics. We tend to develop them prematurely, but with again proper surgery in concert with great blood-sugar management, they can be easily spotted and corrected.

The last, but not least problem with all people, not just diabetics is glaucoma. This disease cause damage to the eye by the raising of the ocular (internal) pressure within the eye.

There are few things beyond good control that can prevent glaucoma, except one. Extract of cannabis. There is great research and development of non-psychoactive cannabis oil and cannabis seed oil. Hopefully these products will be available to legally use soon.

Please support these efforts. They do not make a person "high".

They lower the pressure in the eye and retard growth of unwanted blood vessels. This is accomplished naturally, not through pharmaceuticals.

Make sure to have your child's vision checked every year, or if they have a brittle condition, every half-year. Furthermore, these check-ups should be done by an ophthalmologist, not an optician.

Question: What special care should I take with my diabetic child and dental health?

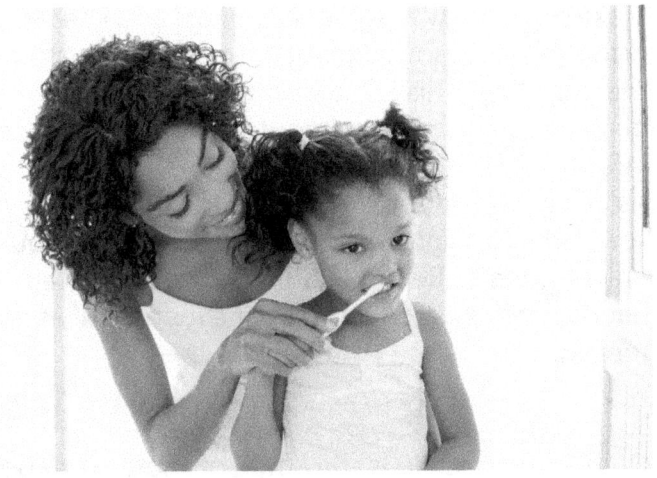

Answer: Diabetes affects the level of sugar in the blood-stream and all other bodily fluids. Saliva being just one. Dry-mouth is a constant problem for diabetics. It creates in the mouth a high degree of decay causing acids to form. Saliva keeps the PH balance normal and the absence of it can weaken teeth and inflame gum tissues. Another good reason to drink plenty of water and to stay hydrated. Plenty of water before sleeping is recommended and a mouth-rinse that can protect the teeth from the effects of dry-mouth. This is in addition to brushing and flossing, everyday. A water jet flossing device is highly recommended to not just remove food from between teeth, but to message the gum tissues as well. Hopefully, your child will have a low-sugar diet and this will lesson the damage to their teeth which normal sugar consumption would have caused.

Make sure to have regular cleanings and check-ups, including ultra-sound plaque removal from around the gum-line. This is the best way to remove bacteria build-up in the mouth and and minimize infection of the gums.
As always, do your best to avoid infections of any sort through hygiene and avoidance of infectious environments. Remind your child to wash their hands and avoid touching their eyes as well as their mouth.

Question: My child is still afraid of shots. How do I remove this fear and make them calm?

Answer: Many people of all ages are afraid or have an aversion to hypodermic shots. This is, I believe, instilled in us as a conditioned response. We have a distant memory of the pain from shots and the smell of the alcohol activates this cellular memory and we tense up and feel pain that isn't there. All based on the response of smell and the great amount of emotional recall it triggers.
Remind yourself and then your child that the shot they had that hurt so much wasn't an insulin injection, but a booster shot or some other type of shot that caused all that pain. Show them that it doesn't hurt by being the best injector in the world and encouraging them to inject themselves. If you are afraid, then they will be too. Even inject yourself

with an empty syringe, if needed. Dis-associate pain from the injection formula and replace it with routine. The "pain" is in their mind.

Again, send your child to a great diabetic camp or clinic immediately after a diagnosis. Become proficient in preparing their shot(s). My mom was so good at injecting me , I just stayed in bed and she injected me in my half-sleep. This may also help in the beginning.

Question: What items should my JD child have with them at all times?

Answer: They should have their "diabetic survival kit". It should have a syringe with a small amount of fast acting insulin, sugary items to stave off insulin reactions, their blood testing kit and a emergency shot of glucagon.

These items should always accompany your child everywhere they go. To school, to church, the mall, or anywhere else.

When your child is first diagnosed with diabetes and they are of school age, have a sit down with all their teachers and discuss your child's needs.

Do not assume they understand the condition. Bring them up to speed and insist that they observe your child and monitor their condition. They need to be able to spot low blood-sugars as well as you can.

Also, your teachers must be prepared to administer the glucagon shot if your child goes into unconsciousness and cannot be revived with oral glucose.

At least have the school nurse trained and able to respond if a serious blood-sugar issue arises. My teachers knew about my condition and we had sugary snacks in the classroom for such occasions.

Question: Can my JD child stay overnight at friend's houses?

Answer: Yes, there should be no restrictions, IF your child is stable and can administer their own insulin injections and blood testing. Obviously the parents need to be informed and educated in JD so they can understand the situation and respond. Also, ask the parents to not feed your child foods that are restricted and especially, deserts.

Question: What is the normal range for blood-sugars?

Answer: Before eating the reading should be as close to 90 (90 milligrams per deciliter, or mg /dl. The range for a normal person is 85-140 mg/dl. A normal person one hour after eating should not exceed 150.

As a diabetic, you must lower your "set point'" or the blood-sugar level in which your brain starts to shout,"feed me!"

If your child is in poor control then this set point is high (120-140). As they gain better control this should get back to normal or, 85 - 100 mg/dl before they "need" to eat.

After eating, their blood sugar should not exceed 160 for too long. This is why exercise and movement after eating is so essential for a JD. It slows down the digestion by causing the blood not to concentrate in the digestive system, but to circulate throughout the muscles of the body.

Better still, the exercise they get also lowers their blood sugar which balances out the process for a stable, working metabolism.

After two hours the blood-sugar level should be back in the normal (non-diabetic) level of 110- 130 mg/dl.

Some people start to have mild symptoms of low blood-sugar at 80-90. If the blood-sugar is below 70, it is an insulin reaction.

If you cannot confirm an insulin reaction by not having a testing kit, assume it is a reaction and treat it as previously described earlier in the book.

Question: Why are diabetics more prone to illness?

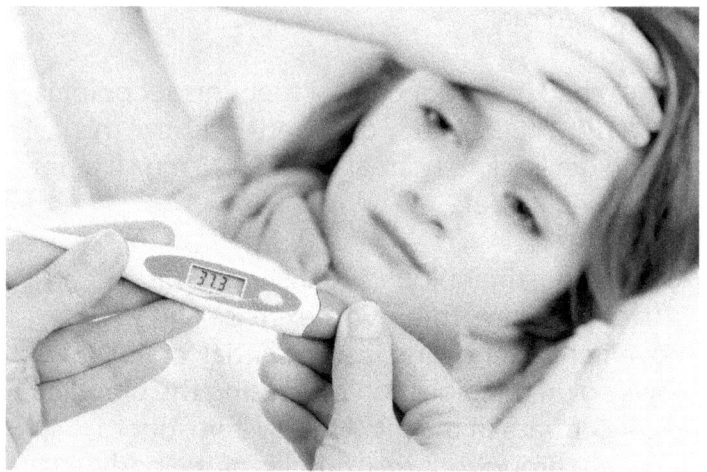

Answer: Because diabetes in both of it's types, is an auto-immune condition. The immune system for diabetics has been compromised and this makes us susceptible to every cold, virus or allergy going around. All caution must be maintained to avoid exposure to these conditions and the bacteria/germs that cause them. Make sure you JD child washes their hands and keeps their feet clean as well. Ingrown nails can become infected, so always cut them straight across the nail and not in a rounded manner. Check your child's feet for cuts or abrasions and always have your child wear shoes with clean socks. Make sure the shoes are not ill-fitting.

Furthermore, have all your child's inoculations, especially flu shots done as directed by your doctor, New research has shown that diabetics need to receive hepatitis B shots as well.

Fortify your child's immune system at all turns.

Question: What do I do if my child gets sick? Are there special actions to take?

Answer: If your child has a cold and is sedentary most of the day, then they will need more insulin than normal. Anytime your diabetic child is in a situation where they have restricted movement or activity also requires extra amounts of insulin. Most importantly, any kind of infection or flu will require extra insulin to counter the effects of the infection raising blood-sugars along with lack of normal exorcize. It is also best to again, curtail carbohydrates, especially sugars which help to feed the fever from infections or sickness. Your diabetic child probably will need very little food if they are resting or sleeping most of the day, yet they will need more insulin, even with less food intake. Check your child's blood-sugars and don't forget to give them lots of water. Both to hydrate and help flush impurities, but to also assist removing the extra sugar from the body, that are eliminated via the kidneys.

Question: If my child has very high blood-sugar because of illness or any reason, what should I do?

Answer: One, give them a shot of short acting insulin. Two, as mentioned above, give them lots of water too help "flush" the extra sugar from the body and three, have them rest and NOT exercise at all. When the bloodstream is full of glucose and there is no appreciable amount of insulin, the body cannot metabolize at all and the cells, again, cannot open to receive oxygen and remove carbon dioxide. Thus, exercising would only result in a build-up of lactic acid and other toxins that do not improve the situation. It worsens it. The best way to lower very high blood-sugars is to allow the body to return to an acceptable level of insulin to start proper metabolism. Only then will exercise act to lower blood-sugars.

Question: Is there a cure yet for Juvenal diabetes?

Answer: Yes and no. There has been widening success with pancreatic transplants, but they are invasive and very costly, involving years of anti-rejection drug regimens. These procedures are usually accompanied by kidney transplants as well. They do not fully restore a person back to total health, but are working as long as there is no organ rejection.

The real answer lies in replacing the beta cell in the pancreas without replacing the total organ. The beta cells produce insulin and regulate the insulin level in the body. This, I believe, is the best way to "cure" JD. The research in genetics is eventually the answer, in gene splicing or even growing new pancreases in a lab.

We were told many years ago that there would be a cure within "just a few years". It is beyond high time for creating a genetic cure for diabetes, of both types. The amount of cost, grief and suffering that would be spared is incalculable. This should be a national priority. Please do what you can to make it so.

Question: What about insulin pumps? Aren't they a cure?

Answer: No, They are not a cure, they are just a different insulin delivery system. It doesn't "cure" anything. They simply inject insulin by an electrical pump and regulate blood sugars to release insulin when needed. In my opinion, these devices are getting over prescribed. They are for people with extremely brittle conditions who cannot regulate their blood-sugars without them. This is a very small percentage of people with JD. If the largest percentage of people did what I have advocated in this book, they would not require insulin pumps at all. They should one, get their JD in control and two, take multiple shots during the day. Just about everyone as they get older require more insulin during the day and night. I take an injection in the morning and before every meal, or when needed.

Most people would not consider having a device sticking into their body attached to electric pump as desirable.

We need a cure, folks, not a fix.

Question: What kinds of insulin should my child use?

Answer: Your doctor would make that determination, but two types, short and long lasting insulins are usually prescribed. Both types are taken as a morning shot. Then a short lasting insulin, if needed, as a "night shot". Or, if an extremely brittle condition, before every meal.

The ideal pattern is to have an overlap of insulin so that high blood-sugar can be averted. The younger and thus, smaller child, will probably only require a morning shot.

Question: Where is the best place to give an insulin injection?

Answer: The back of the arm is best if you inject for them. Remember to rotate the injections from the right arm to the left and also to change the injection site, as well.

If they inject themselves, then the upper leg of the thigh is best. For the fastest injection response, they can inject the abdomen, which is closer to the heart.

Question: What is diabetic camp?

Answer: Diabetic camps are usually held in the summer to train your child in the mechanics of being a diabetic.How to draw insulin. How to inject themselves and all the other things they will need to know to master this condition. better still, your child will be around other diabetic children, possibly for the first time. They can relate to others and the others can relate to your child. This also helps to "normalize" their diabetes, by being around just other diabetics and see that their lives are focused on being kids that have diabetes, other than being diabetic children.

Diabetic camp is where many of these kids learn what "exercise" means. They keep these kids active all day and night and give them tight control. Hopefully, this becomes a habit for the rest of their lives. I attended diabetic camp for 8 years and met many other people with diabetes who I became friends with.

Question: Should I buy special diabetic foods or prepared meals?

Answer: No. There is a whole industry dedicated to selling you prepared meals. These are low sugar and low fat with an emphasis on low calories. They also taste like cardboard.

Please learn to cook. For your child and for yourself, along with the whole rest of the family. You can make great tasting meals with plenty of nutrition, quickly and easily. The main component of taste comes from fats, which are not restricted in our diet. The principal reason diet food tastes so bad is basic lack of fats.

An example would be stews. Meat combined with plenty of vegetables slowly cooked in a crock pot with the natural fats is loaded with not just great taste and satisfying substance, but is also, low in carbohydrate and perfectly within what we are striving for.

A balanced diet for a diabetic, without stripping away all of the pleasure of eating.

As a parent, you will find yourself besieged with hidden sugar in the foods you buy at the supermarket. Innocuous items such as ketchup, mayonnaise and most baked foods are packed with sugar. The most damaging of all the sweeteners used (and abused) is high fructose corn syrup (HFCS). It is in just about everything and you need to run from it. It is, in my opinion, the most addictive sweetener ever put on the market. It's quite true that table sugar (sucrose) has no nutritional value other than straight carbohydrate, but even so, it's still a food. HFCS is not a food, it is a chemical. A by-product of corn. It mimics sugar but does not digest the same and is intensely habit forming in that it promoted more consumption to maintain that level of chemical in the body and to keep the person on the blood-sugar roller-coaster. The shocking level of obesity recorded in the last 25 years parallels the increased use of this chemical in our food supply, thus, making our pallet crave more sweetness than necessary.

This creates a problem that all diabetics must change; the level of sweetness that you have in your mouth and learning to accept less.

The better your child's diet is followed, the more "sugar sensitive" they become and they will not crave junk food and trashy high-sugar, high salt snacks. Those foods will eventually taste like poison in their mouths. The reaction all people have when weened off of excess sugar and salt.

Don't discount the abuse of sodium and salts as well. They are bad for blood pressure and retention of fluids in the body.

By cooking for yourself, you can control these factors directly. Back to ketchup and mayonnaise. You can make them both yourself without adding sugar or corn syrup. Use salsa instead of ketchup. Watch for the hidden sugar and start weening your child off of "The White Horse".

Another word of caution. Do not try to eliminate all the sugars in your child's diet overnight. The drastic change can trigger heart and mental issues due to hypoglycemia. Gradually work to reduce extra sugars and salts and transition in steps toward better control. In six months of reduced exposure to "normal" foods, your diabetic child won't be able to eat fast food french fries the same. They will brush off all the salt and the ketchup will taste like tomato flavored syrup. The unhealthy spike in blood-sugar from the starch won't be welcome anymore, either.

The great dividend of cooking and preparing your child's meals will be evident when your child avoids "bad" foods because they no longer crave them. They become accustomed to good food and crave them instead.

Question: How do i measure my JD child's health other than blood-sugar levels?

Answer: The best indication of great control is through a hemoglobin test of the blood, done usually once or twice a year. It measure how much glucose is in the red blood cells. It is referred to as an H1C test and is rated by percentage numbers. The lower the number the better. A diabetic should strive to get to 7% or below. Above 8% and there is strong indication for complications from their diabetes because of long and short range blood-sugar control issues. So, to put this books' intent in a nutshell; lack of control insures complications and control prevents or at least, keeps them to a minimum. The red blood cells regenerate every 90 days or so and this allows the level of glucose in the these cells to diminish through better control. At the sake of reiteration, follow the advise of this book and you can keep this crucial indication of diabetic health under control and prevent complications.

Question: How do I reduce insulin resistance?

Answer: By a liver cleanse. By removing as many carbohydrates as possible from their diet and restricting the calories taken in, the liver will empty itself of the glucose stored there. People with insulin resistance have far too much glucose stored in their livers and it is released into the bloodstream to make room for even more glucose. A vicious cycle. To break this cycle, force the body to give up it's extra stored energy. If your child is insulin resistant, allow them to have mild insulin reactions and under-treat them as far as low blood sugar is concerned.

An apple to an insulin resistant person is all the sugar the person can tolerate and the liver will kick in the remaining glucose by hormonal response. If you had treated the insulin reaction normally, with sugary items like candy, it would have treated the reaction, but spiked the person's blood-sugar sky high in the process. This cleanse must be accompanied by constant blood-sugar testing and lots of hydration to help remove the extra sugar being vacated from the body.

When a person's insulin is working properly, that person can feel the effects of low blood-sugar come on strongly at meal times, because of having a demonstrable lack of extra stored glucose to "kick in". This means with proper control your insulin doses can decrease and with it, your extra weight. The other factor that I mentioned previously, that contributes to insulin resistance.

If your child is an athlete, remember they are now 'brittle' when it comes to low blood-sugars. They have little, if any reserves of available glucose and they will hit The "sugar wall" very hard and very fast. This is normal, because you have substituted stored energy from body fat and glucose in the liver, to active use of food energy and a marked increase in the body's metabolism. A conditioned diabetic athlete can tolerate far more carbohydrate then a non athletic diabetic because they can actually "cope" with these foods. Why? No insulin resistance.

Question: What changes with adolescence?

Answer: Everything.

The constant growing and hormonal turmoil alone is hard enough to deal with as a normal teenagers but with Juvenal diabetes all the factors are intensified. First, the growing spurts that start require more food and sleep to build new tissues in the body. Plus, your JD adolescent naturally will be larger and heavier, thus, requiring more insulin as well. This is completely normal. All children require more insulin as they grow.

Hormonally, they will have adjustments to make to insulin or foods as these levels of hormones increase and they start to take on adult growth characteristics. The amount of food along with insulin must increase in line with these increases in maturity. Don't be discouraged if your JD child requires an additional shot or shots. This is what happens with an increase in muscle mass and not because of insulin resistance.

The changes in emotional stability can be a cause of stress which, of course, creates elevated sugars. Starting your diabetic child on the right path as pre-adolescents helps immensely in helping them exercise discipline and control as adolescents.

Question: The idea of limited carbohydrates isn't going to be easy to do. How do I accomplish this without making my JD child feel deprived?

Answer: Food psychology. If Friday night is spaghetti and meat-ball night in your house-hold and it's a tradition that makes the whole family happy, you don't have to stop this tradition. Just change it.

If, for instance, your fourteen year old son would have 3 cups of pasta with endless sauce with meat-balls smothered in melted cheese. Those days must stop. Instead make larger meat-balls stuffed with vegetables, that sit on top of one cup of pasta and limited cheese, perhaps parmesan cheese or feta, instead of cheddar. Skip the garlic toast unless your child is active and you have a very satisfying meal with all the same components as usual, but in healthy portions. As a way of keeping that good feeling going and not letting your child feel deprived, serve them some leftover spaghetti and meat balls for lunch the next day (just them) and you both will feel good about spaghetti night.

Also, try to serve sandwiches open faced, with one piece of bread on the bottom instead of two pieces. The single piece of bread is 100 calories of carbohydrate, which spikes your child's insulin needs. Give them plenty of food to put on the sandwich and they will be more than satisfied with less starch. You can fold the bread over and make a thicker sandwich, if they want something to have in their hand. Three pieces of bread, over three meals, that might have been eaten that day can now be dedicated to eating a better source of carbohydrate such as vegetables or fruit.

Question: Is it safe to eat all that protein and fat? Isn't this like a Dr. Atkins type of diet?

Answer: By varying the types of protein, both animal and vegetable, a person gets good long lasting food energy. Saturated fats that are high in beef are only a limited food option and as I mentioned earlier, should be a non-staple.

Fats are very good for you and slow down the assimilation of carbohydrates. Also it is not difficult to eat a large input of calories with very little actual fat, due to the fact that fats have 9 calories per gram as apposed to 7 calories per gram for carbohydrates or proteins.

Using a pat of butter to make your scrambled eggs may make some misguided people wince, but consistent evidence shows that butter is FAR better for a person than margarine, or any butter substitute. It doesn't mean everything you cook should swim in butter, but using artificial anything, be it sweeteners or flavors or fats, is bad for you. Using olive oil and other, non-saturated, low cholesterol producing oils are high on the list of fats in our diabetic diet. Trans-fats are not on our diet.

As I've said repeatably, baked goods are not a staple for your JD child, so lard and shortening is not an issue. Our diet is low in dairy, so fat from milk, cheese and cream is at a minimum already and are not a food issue. Tropical oils such as palm and coconut oils are avoided naturally because our diet is very low on refined and processed snacks. Also, because of our low starch approach, deep frying is also at a minimum and a treat, never a staple food type. So, the two items on the saturated fat list are there: butter and meat. But, neither one must be used for every meal or everyday, as well.

Forty plus years ago the book The Doctor Adkins Diet Revolution was published and it shook up the dieting community by advocating a protein and fats diet, with NO carbohydrates at all. This was only intended for obese people and is not a healthy or sustainable diet. A no carbohydrate diet causes the body cannibalize itself quickly and floods the blood stream with ketones, the poison from this process. This is the precursor to keto-acidosis. To say the very least, completely wrong for a diabetic. My father used this system and it only led to gout and a yo-yo effect to his weight. As soon as he re-introduced any carbohydrates to his diet, the weight returned. I was amazed when my father used my urine testing strips to test his own urine and he rejoiced when he saw that he was producing ketones. Proof that he was cannibalizing himself and producing poison. Simply wrong.

I described a liver cleanse with little or no carbohydrates, but that was to battle insulin resistance and not a diet. Limit the carbohydrates, but don't stop them unless your child is extremely brittle and a doctor recommends it.

Diet fads and diabetes never mix. Please do what I've described in this book and see the positive results.

I say again that I am not a doctor, but I reject the findings of certain diabetic advocacy groups. They stress far too much carbohydrate and dairy consumption and most egregiously, attack the general use of nutritious fats.

I saw the food graph for the top JD diabetic advocacy group and it broke down the percentage of foods as one quarter proteins, one quarter carbohydrates and HALF of the rest, vegetables, which of course, are carbohydrate! No provision for fruit or fats at all. Plus, they added an extra serving item, a dinner roll as well. Straight carbohydrate. The vegetables as shown on the plate illustration graph showed half of the vegetables as baby carrots. Carrots are the vegetable highest on the glycemic index. They are basically fruit.

So, this reputable diabetes organization advocates a diet for diabetics which is actually by the example given, over 70% carbohydrate, not the stated 25%.

I would please ask you for a bit of faith in the directives I give in this book. It is just my advise. But I serve no other master than the truth. If you tried following the other folks diet and advise and it didn't work and your JD child is still depressed, obese and insulin resistant. Then please try what I have been advocating and see for yourself.

Chapter 6
The Conclusion

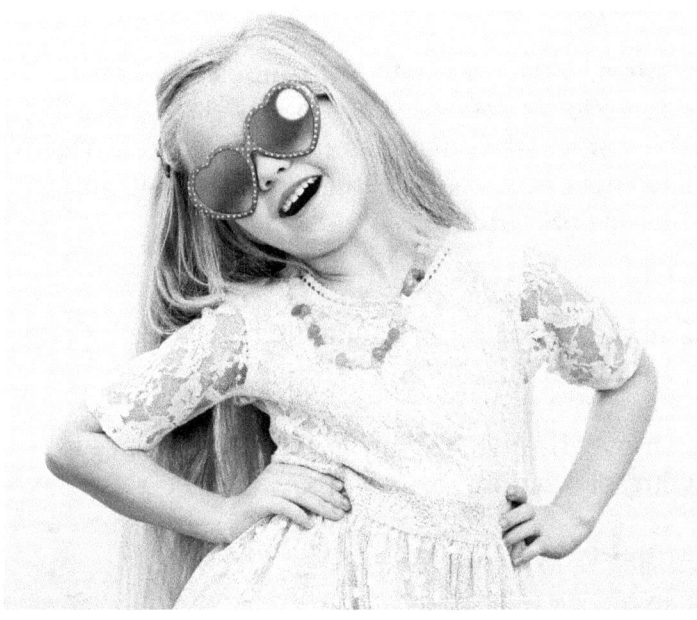

I hope that this book, as brief and concise as it is written, will be of help to you and your diabetic child. Please try the things that I have prescribed for your child and see for yourself that my diet and exercise advice will work wonders.

So lets review.

Good blood-sugar control is the key to good diabetic control. This is obtained through a high protein/fat, low carbohydrate diet with plenty of supplements and water. Activity after every meal and stress reduction through exercise and social interaction. Mix with plenty of rest and sleep and you and your child are on your way to defeating The Triangle of Despair.

Instead, you have created the opposite. When depression is defeated and obesity eliminated, the only corner left is diabetes and with it's control, you have now, replaced The Triangle of Despair with The Triangle of Triumph.

Diabetes is again, not your fault, but, it needs to be your cause.

Remove the guilt, shame and fear and replace it with solid action.

My best to you and yours.

About the author

Sean M. Kinkaid,is a freelance writer and teacher living in Portland, Oregon.

www.ingramcontent.com/pod-product-compliance
Lightning Source LLC
Chambersburg PA
CBHW070935180526
45168CB00003B/1091